One Day at a Time

One Day at a Time

By Warren Evans

To order additional copies of this book, contact:
The Augusta Free Press, Publishing Division
www.augustafreepress.com
sales@augustafreepress.com

Acknowledgements

Four outstanding physicians: Phillips R. Bryan Jr., M.D., Stefan M. Gorsch, M.D., Charles R. Pauly, M.D., William Toomy, M.D. Each is a leader in his field of specialty. Without their guidance, expertise, and kind assistance this book would NEVER have been possible.

Incidentally, much credit must be also given their cheerful, accommodating, and efficient staffs.

* * *

To all the wonderful people that have been in my life during these past three years I express my gratitude.

Other books by Warren Evans

CHINA - THE RETURN OF MARCO POLO
VIRGINIA: THE WESTERN HIGHLANDS
RED LEAF 645
THE CORPSE MOWS AT MIDNIGHT
MARVELOUS MAGGIE

In Memory
of
Tim McDow

Who was unable to complete his
journey on the Big "C" Line.

A NOTE FROM THE AUTHOR: As you read the book, you will note that I have chosen a capital letter as the name for each character. Sometimes, for clarity, I have appended to the capital a number or another letter.

As you get along further in the book you may note that a second character may have the same capital letter as one earlier in the story. Be not dismayed. After all, in real life, most of our names are used by other individuals.

Prologue

I turned 80 recently (2 August 2003).

So, what's the big deal? You ask.

In response, I would say that I'm just as anxious to hold on to life as a kid in his 40s. It is because I believe that a preponderance of readers feel the same way that I write this monograph.

I truly hope this report about my ongoing three year *Voyage On The Big "C" Line* between the mythical ports of REFRACTORY and REFLECTION will help someone.

If one reader derives one thing from this writing, to make for a better life, then it has all been worthwhile.

[UNEXPECTED NOTE: Two months work and 20,000 words just crashed last night - and I didn't have a back-up. So, now you KNOW that my starting over from scratch should tell you something. It should tell you that I'm irrevocably committed to getting this message across to you, the readers.]

Chapter 1   *In the Beginning*

It was exactly three years ago. I was experiencing bothersome problems with my plumbing system. It was very annoying, so much so, that I decided to visit Dr. T. In addition to being a friend he is an internist and my long time primary care physician.

A number of tests were performed upon me. One of them was the Prostatic Specific Antigen (PSA) test. This is given to prostate cancer candidates. An elevated count generally indicates that there is a high probability of prostate cancer being present.

In my case the PSA count was exceedingly low. It was so low that the chances of my having prostate cancer were very remote.

I was now in the treatment room with my friend and doctor. I must explain something to you. Nothing could take place medically until he fully reviewed the prospects for the nearby university's basketball team. We both supported that team. He, himself, had been an outstanding college point guard at another school.

Suddenly, the mood in the examining room changed. He put on his sterile gloves and bade me to drop my trousers. He was about to perform a digital examination.

It was very prolonged (by my estimation). The probing and maneuvering of his digit was accompanied by
a few *hmms.*

"Okay," he eventually said. "Get dressed and come
back to the office." He then stepped out of the room,
closing the door behind him. I was certain that we
would not be talking about basketball.

When I stepped into his office he was dictating
something into a machine. He waved me into a chair
without missing a beat of his dictation.

"I'm sending you to Dr. B. He's a great urologist,
and I know that you'll like him." There was some small
talk and then he continued with the subject at hand.
"When I did the digital I was not at all comfortable with
what I felt. I'd like Dr. B. to take it from here.

"He's a good man that really knows what he's
doing." No question, but my buddy, Dr. T. was selling
me a bill of goods. "You'll really like him. While you
were getting dressed I set up an appointment with him
for you."

At that point in time, the last thing on my mind was
basketball. My friend was mumbling something about
needing "a big man."

I made a hasty retreat.

I was very apprehensive as to what would happen next.

Chapter 2   *Visit to the Plumber*

The waiting room for the Urology group was virtually filled to capacity. With several exceptions, we were all males. I assumed that the ladies present were there to accompany their spouses. It was, then, that I concluded that urologists would starve to death if they had to depend upon the *weaker sex* for their business.

After filling out forms and signing more forms I settled down in a chair awaiting the summons from Dr. B.'s nurse.

Nurses were coming to the door every few minutes summoning a patient for a specific urologist. I sighed with relief each time.

You must understand my frame of mind at that time. I was not enamored with anything that was taking place.

"Mr. Evans," called the smiling nurse standing by the open door.

I awakened from my reverie and followed her into the treatment room. She asked me a few questions. My answers were duly logged into the file that she carried. She then advised me that Dr. B. would be in shortly.

After some minutes, I heard a rapping on the door.

"Come in," I said.

The door opened and a very mild-mannered doctor entered. We shook hands, exchanged a few pleasantries.

I advised him of my complaints. He asked a few questions which I answered. He then told me to get on the table. After some few minutes of probing and whatever else that urologists do he repeated the examination that I received from Dr. T.

Some time and some place, along the way, I had X-rays taken of me that he was now scoping.

He confirmed the suspicion offered by Dr. T. He then explained that he was referring me to radiation oncologists at a cancer hospital in a neighboring city.

Incidentally, he assured me that they were great.

By now, I had formed the opinion that the doctor's union had invoked *the big build up routine* as a prerequisite for a pass-off to another doctor.

*   *   *

The very next Monday I drove the 30 miles to the cancer clinic. It was part of the hospital in a city to the north of mine.

The waiting room was doing a land office business. I reported directly to an admitting clerk that supervised the traditional *new boy initiation*. After filling out forms and answering questions I moved back to the waiting area to an empty chair.

I heard my name being called. Standing by an open door was a middle age lady. She had a delightful smile. She offered a quick comment on what a wonderful fall day we had.

Before I knew it, we had reached a nursing station

where a cute little blonde awaited me. I followed her into a darkened room. There were several chairs against a wall. She suggested I leave my jacket there. She then directed me to the very large machine and table in the center of the room.

Once mounted upon the table she commenced taking various measurements. She had me move into specific positions. She explained that she would be taking some pictures. In addition, she would be arranging the set-up for my radiation treatment. I would not be receiving any until the following day.

Come the next day, I was back at the same place at the same time. I was told that the treatment would be a five-day-a-week thing (or maybe it was four days - senior memory problem) For the sake of convenience let us just assume that it was a daily thing.

Without being coached I placed my jacket on the chair and mounted the table. A few more measurements were taken by the technician - it was another young lady. I was very impressed by the extreme warmth and friendliness of the nurses and techs that had taken care of me during the past days. It made me feel like family.

The technician took a few measurements. She then gave me a brief explanation of what I could expect. She then walked to the end of the darkened room where a control room was located. She entered it. It would be from there that she would regulate the radiation equipment.

From my perspective there is very little to report on the radiation procedure, itself. Much water has gone under the bridge since my radiation. I would say that the actual radiation session took approximately 45 minutes. It was painless and involved no effort on my part. The technician made certain that the radiation machine concentrated on the predetermined target areas of my body.

Once every week I would have a visit with a radiation oncologist. It was either Dr. K., head of the radiation department, or another physician. Dr. K. sported a trim van dyke beard. I figured the personable doc to be in his late 40s or early 50s. (Did I tell you that I'm lousy estimating ages?). The majority of the time I would meet with his younger associate, Dr. M. I pegged him at being 10 years younger than his boss. He had a great sense of humor.

I was highly impressed with all of the personnel that I came in contact with from that department. They were, in every way, a friendly group that always treated me as a close relative (on good terms).

Upon completion of my cycle of radiation I was passed back to Dr. B. It may seem weird but irrespective of a daily 60-mile drive, I felt sad at the prospect of leaving those very wonderful people.

As I recall, my treatment went on for about six months. Neither the driving nor the treatment, itself, created problems for me. It was my stomach that took the beating. Suffice to say: Each day was an adventure for me insofar as my GI system was concerned. As I think back on those days that was my only side effect.

Chapter 3   *Out of the Woodwork*

At this juncture let me point out that I live at home with only my little Westie, Winkie.

I have three married children. The oldest, a boy, lives with his wife and their two children in the northern part of this state. He is a teacher.

To the south of me, also within the state, is my married daughter. She and her husband have two dogs - no children. She is also a teacher.

The youngest, a boy, lives two-thirds across the country from me. He, too, is married. He and his wife have a cat. He works in the travel industry.

So, with no family, at hand, you might think that I am isolated. But, such is not the case.

From, literally, *out of the woodwork* I have found myself surrounded by supportive friends that I never knew I had.

Let me be quick to tell you that I did not, to the best of my recollection, tell anybody about my disease, *The Big "C."* (Maybe I told one or two people). The point is that I never made a public announcement concerning my health. You must understand that all through my life I have always been very independent and SELF sufficient.

And another thing! I really believe that I was ashamed and embarrassed at being diagnosed as having cancer. Honestly and truly, I did not want anybody to know that I was afflicted with that disease.

That was all to change.

It began with my church where I serve as an usher. One of my fellow ushers, G., some 15 years younger than me, had recently lost his wife to cancer. During her illness he dedicated every waking (and some sleeping ones, I would surmise) to her care.

He is one of those rare souls that has never been heard to say an unkind word about anybody else. What is equally unusual, is that nobody has ever said an unkind word about him. G. is a very mild-mannered individual that I'm certain would do anything for me.

Like osmosis, we have bonded into a friendship. It is unlike any that I have ever experienced in my life. It started when he first learned about my health (obviously, I had informed him about my condition).

He calls me virtually each day. We attend athletic events together. We frequently eat out together. He's got three married children with kids of their own. I'm so flattered to be constantly invited to their family events.

I'm pleased to report that in my own family, G., is considered a member of ours.

What's so weird is that G. and myself have so little in common. We come from different parts of the country - we did different type work - had different extracurricular interests. Be that as it may, you could not ask for two better friends. I owe so much to him. I find it difficult to envision what it would be like without him by my side.

*   *   *

This young man, D., doesn't go to my church. He's in law enforcement, and I am at least two and one half times as old as him. He's married with three very active youngsters. D. could easily be one of my own children. He'd do anything for me. Nonetheless, at times, his actions can be very frustrating.

His beautiful wife, D2, has proven to be a great friend. By day, she efficiently handles her administrative job. Once the sun falls, she goes back to being mother and homemaker. She's always made me welcome in their home.

Her greatest contribution to my welfare was putting me in touch with her mom and pop, F&G. Their home is in another part of the state. F. is a recovering cancer patient. Upon hearing of my plight she sent me a lengthy and detailed primer. A compendium of instructions telling me how to address my illness. When I passed it on to my oncologist, Dr. G., he observed that I couldn't go wrong following it and suggested that I run with it.

*　　*　　*

From my church many people come to mind. I'd start with a handsome and youthful looking couple, S&E. They're retirees that moved here for their retirement from the Midwest. In the four years, or so, that I've known them they've always taken the same seats in church. They fall within the purview of my ushering *talents*. They're warm, friendly, and endowed with wonderful frames of mind.

I can recall when E (Mr.) was fighting his own war against cancer. His full head of hair was rapidly disappearing. It wasn't long before he arrived at church with a glossy and shiny scalp - 100 percent bald. In my former insensitive persona, I teased him. He would grin and good naturedly respond. In the weeks to come we would continue our bantering.

Then came the day - his hair began peeping through *the cracks*. It was not long before all of his hair returned.

Oh! how I admired them both for the way in which they handled E.'s serious health problem. If only I could have been supportive of him during that period.

Now, the shoe is on the other foot. He's in remission, and I am fighting the *battle*.

The support they give me is continuous and constant. It recharges me with each and every supportive contact. At a minimum, it is no fewer than one per week. They'll send humorous greeting cards. On a weekly basis they send chatty e-mails that report their week's activity. At the same time they ask about mine. Always, they encourage me to pursue to completion all that I undertake.

They always greet me with a smile along with warm handshakes. S&E are so supportive. The waves that I encounter are not so rough because of them.

*   *   *

Then there are the very wonderful ladies, J&ML. They are sisters that have chosen not to marry. They live together and share a wonderful life through the many acts of kindness that they heap upon those around them.

On a very regular basis they send me greeting cards that often are spiritual or inspirational. From time to time they will call me - just to see how I'm doing. Always they ask me how they can help me.

They forever look for unique knick-knacks or *whatever* that they think I might like. It will come to me as a surprise gift accompanied by a wonderful greeting card. The latest gift to come to me with a greeting card was a very colorful tie. It contained, in living color, many of the world's flags. J&ML knew that I had spent more than 30 years in the travel business with much time spent traveling the many countries represented on the tie.

How they knew that flags have always been a fetish of mine. Within 10 minutes of receiving the tie I had ID'd the nationality for each flag. I'm never content to allow a flag to go unidentified.

Yes, the sisters J&ML, through smiles, encouragement, and generosity are very definitely a part in my healing therapy.

*　　*　　*

Then there is G. She is a fellow usher at church. As a gentleman, I would not venture to guesstimate her age. Suffice to say, that she is older than 65. No matter her years of a very full life she still remains a very active and caring woman.

Since the very onset of my illness she has never ceased to display concern for my condition. On those occasions on which I offered complaints about myself she would counter by offering practical curative steps.

G&J, her husband, moved here a number of years ago. He had retired from a career of public service in their native New Jersey.

Subsequent to their arrival here he became seriously ill. He was to become very dependent upon G. Though,

I would not see him at church services I would see him at church socials. He and G. would always save a place for me at their table.

He was gifted in working with his hands and was blessed with an Irish sense of humor. He never left you in doubt as to what his position might be. I always enjoyed it when he was in a *tell it as it is* mode. He was always fun to be around.

As the days went by his condition deteriorated. Less than a year ago, J. died. During his illness, G. was constantly by his side. She was a very faithful and caring spouse to the very end. Even, unto death, G. will to this day, express her love for him through devout and loving prayer.

To me, she has shown caring and concern. I feel that knowing her has made me a better person.

Her caring has also included a 90-year-old woman, a fellow parishioner, who subsequently became home-bound. Up until the time of her recent death, G. was very attentive to all of her needs and wants.

G. is a very special person that has touched many lives in a very loving way.

*   *   *

Five years my senior is B. He is a stand-tall man who is very much given to being frank. He is another individual who will say it as it is. Some few years ago he became a widow. Just knowing him, seeing him, and fielding that occasional call has meant so much to me. He forever expresses interest on how I feel and how I am getting along.

They may be small acts, but to me, it's the quality

that he expresses to me that makes me think so much about him.

His adult son, R. generally accompanies him to church. More reserved than his father he is in every way equally sincere. It is the smile that he will flash to me that acts upon me as a catharsis on those occasions when I may be *down.*

Then there is P. (R.'s wife). She does not attend church. I first came in contact with her at the fitness center that I attend. She, too, has always expressed great interest and concern for me. I can count on her if the need should arise.

It's a very wonderful family.

* * *

Then, there is the very prolific P. family. There is husband, wife, three daughters and two sons. I have known them for many years. Since the onset of my illness, I know that their prayers on my behalf have been constant. I am forever running into the family matriarch at either church or at the fitness center. She is never too rushed to patiently inquire about my updated situation. She will also bring me up to date on the comings and goings of her far flung off-spring.

How wonderful it is to know that this wonderful family has time in their busy lives for me.

* * *

V. and R. are concerned neighbors. V. never ceases to express concern for my day-to-day condition. She constantly urges me to notify her immediately if some emergency should arise. It should be noted that she, herself, is a cancer survivor in remission.

I would also like to point out that she constantly cares for her husband, R., a recent leg amputee, who has been undergoing a very difficult rehabilitative program.

* * *

L., T., J., D. - What a wonderful family. L. just called and asked if I would mind if she dropped by with some ham biscuits (timing is perfect, it's dinner time).

Talk about kismet - I had just commenced writing about this family when the call came. L., the wife, and J., the pretty teenager, are forever inquiring about my welfare. D., the son, is off to college.

T., a good friend and business associate, is in his early 50s. He has recently been diagnosed with lung cancer.

* * *

There are so many individuals that I see each week at the same time each week at my church. Their smiles and words of interest and concern have meant so much to me. It makes the act of going to church so fulfilling and so complete.

Dare I mention R&K, M, MA, P&P2, G&A, C&D, T&S?

Well, I have. You may well wonder what purpose it serves in a monograph such as this. Let me address that question.

I truly believe that the interaction with the folks already mentioned plus those that have been inadvertently omitted has served me in many ways.

Thanks to them I have reinforced my mental well being.

I also believe in the efficacy of prayer. I know that I am in their prayers.

It is so uplifting to know that so many wonderful people have reached out to me. Is it any wonder that I am nuturing a better sense of well being.

* * *

Before leaving the trip to my church I can not dismiss the importance of formal spirituality. I believe in God. I'm not particularly devout but I still believe and pray to God. I NEVER try to make my prayers/pleas self serving.

I feel that by including myself, along with the others on my personal prayer list, is the way to go. It has proven to be an effective way to handle my personal petitions.

Our outstanding people oriented pastor, FH, has meant so very much to me. Serving with him is H., an energetic woman with a radiant smile. There is also MA, J, and L that make the church experience joyous for me and my other *brothers and sisters.*

I can not overemphasize the power of God - his workers - and his children in contributing to my present state of being. It's POSITIVELY POWERFUL.

* * *

In my community there is a wonderful support group. It comes under the wing of the American Cancer Society.

The group, itself, is volunteer. It's membership consists of cancer survivors suffering from prostate cancer. They are called *Man To Man of the Valley.*

They publish an informative educational newsletter that is crammed with up-to-the-minute information and news of interest to men with prostate cancer. A typical newsletter contained, among other things: Local news on club activities and local prostate cancer screening schedule.

Monthly club meeting program schedule is high-lighted. Leading medical experts in fields associated with prostate cancer are highlight speakers.

Articles in the newsletter also include nationally released stories on such subjects as diet and legal actions against a pharmaceutical manufacturer. In each article there is a specific connection to prostate cancer. By way of example, the aforementioned legal action was against a manufacturer of a popular drug prescribed to prostate cancer patients.

In addition to the meetings and the newsletter, the group, itself, stands ready to support individual prostate cancer patients when they require assistance.

In communities throughout the nation there are many support groups standing at the ready for cancer patients.

*   *   *

Then there's B., a very attractive woman and local cop, on the fast track. In spite of a busy agenda she can always find the time to look in on me. She has even visited me during hospital stays to see about my needs. A very supportive young lady ever ready to help an old man in time of need.

*   *   *

Always contacting me is my old *back tablemate*, S. For more than two decades we broke bread together at the service club that I had belonged. Always, he and his pretty wife express concern for me. He with booming voice and she with delicate gentility.

*   *   *

Su, whose name I always forget, works out at the wellness center and serves with me on their advisory board. With patented smile she forever inquires as to how I'm getting along. Always, she encourages me to do to completion my ongoing projects.

*   *   *

Then, from the church, is the very pretty and demonstrative T. She and her hubby, M., and their two handsome little boys make a perfect family. I feel so fortunate to have them continually invite me to dine with them on key holidays. It makes me blush (with pleasure) when she showers me with kisses upon my cheeks at church. Believe me! because of T., I feel 30 years younger.

*   *   *

From my church comes the ever persistent won't take NO for an answer T. and his much more relaxed bride N. Together, they always insist that I dine out with them rather than doing a solo at home. I'm fortunate that they take this interest in me.

*   *   *

My voyage on the SS SURVIVOR is not as rough as it would have been without the folks that we have just visited.

Chapter 4 *Detour Along the Way*

Course of radiation over I was now preparing for my next move. It was my understanding that I would now be receiving another form of treatment. If radiation was not successful then other forms of treatment were likely. As I said, it appeared that I would be moving on to the next form of treatment.

I would certainly miss the personnel at the radiation facility. On the other hand, I was happy to be relieved of the drudgery of driving more than 60 miles a day for treatment. I certainly would not miss the unrest that radiation had caused on my stomach.

At that point in time, I had another concern. For some few days I had been experiencing problems with my urinary system. I was of the opinion that the radiation brought it on.

Nonetheless, whether it was the radiation or the cancer, itself, or whatever, causing the malfunction, it had to be corrected. I was particularly concerned with the blockage that caused the malfunction in my *plumbing* system.

I, of course, returned to Dr. B., the urologist.

For the next three months I remained under his care.

During that time he performed certain remedial procedures in the office.

There was also a surgical procedure referred to as a TURP (Transurethal Resection of the Prostate) that he performed upon me as a hospital in-patient.

The following rundown might either help you or a loved one.

I recollect that during the final days of radiation treatment I put up with some very annoying urinary problems. The condition that I was suffering was relieved by the just mentioned surgical procedure, TURP.

What caused my problem was an enlarged (and not cancerous - Benign condition - called BPH (Benign Prostatic Hyperplasia).

The procedure, itself, relieves the blockage around the urinary channel. It further relieves the restricting urethra condition which had impeded the normal flow of urine - suggestive of BPH (Benign Prostatic Hyperplasia).

Now for the typical symptoms. I can assure you that, at one time or another, I was experiencing them all:

(1) Intermittent flow during urination.

(2) Frequent urination because the bladder won't empty.

(3) The feeling that you've never completed urinating. The TURP relieves the blockage.

*   *   *

It was either during the hospital stay for the TURP or another stay (who's counting?) that a very humorous incident took place.

As I recall, I was admitted into the hospital either on Thursday or Friday. Under normal circumstances, I believed that I would have been slated for a Sunday discharge. If memory serves me, the procedure took place on Friday.

There was a big complication.

No, not with the procedure, itself, nor with any unforeseen medical problems.

The complication was that I held two choice season tickets for the nearby university's basketball games. On the Saturday of my stay there was to be, the top home game of the season for me. My alma mater, Missouri University, would be making its first ever visit to the home court of the nearby university. I possessed two prime tickets to the game and because of my hospital confinement, I would be unable to attend the game. If you are a basketball fan, you will agree that IT was a big time complication.

It was about 9 a.m. Saturday morning when the good doctor, in the course of making rounds, paid a visit to me. Dr. B. made a few necessary hand moves upon me. He then pronounced me as coming along very well. He asked me how I was feeling.

I smiled and assured him that I was feeling well.

He then bid me goodbye and proceeded to exit the room.

As he was getting ready to go through the doorway, I called out to him. "Is there any way I could be discharged today so that I can see the game?" After a slight pause I added, "I've got some great seats and would hate to miss it."

In our part of the world it isn't necessary to elaborate as to who would be playing.

Dr. B. had just placed one foot on to the outside corridor floor when he made a sudden stop. He turned around and stepped back into the room.

"You know," he said, "if you were to take your doctor along to the game to watch over you I'm sure something could be worked out."

No problem at all. I had two great seats and good parking. And why not?

Dr. B. then explained that under normal circumstances I would have the catheter removed the following day prior to discharge.

My early discharge would mean wearing the catheter until Monday when it would be removed at Dr. B.'s office.

Whatever it took was good enough for me. I would be going to the big game.

"Well, Warren, you get yourself ready, and I'll arrange for the discharge."

Later that day Dr. B. stopped by my house to pick me up. With parking pass and two choice game tickets, in hand, I hobbled to his car. It was parked behind mine in the driveway.

It was a very short walk. But did I mention that wearing a catheter and moving about was a very prickly affair. Being quite blunt: It's like the inside of your penis is being stuck with pins.

Once settled down in our seats, some 40 minutes later, it all became worthwhile. The band was playing and the students were cheering. Everything was at a fever pitch as we awaited the teams to make their appearance on the court.

Suddenly, Dr. B. looked over at me. "You don't feel well," he observed. Then he added, "You're pale as a ghost."

The good doctor then got up and told me not to worry. He'd be right back. Since, the university had a teaching hospital I was certain that I would become the recipient of some unknown treatment. No doubt he'd return with stretcher bearers to haul me away to the university's nearby hospital.

Some five minutes later he returned holding a large plastic cup. "Here," he handed it to me. "It's Pepsi Cola, drink it. Drink it. It'll make you feel better."

And it did.

There were no more problems. It was a great game that we both thoroughly enjoyed. It was a close game that my alma mater lost. But it was a great game to see.

Immediately following the game Dr. B. delivered me back to the front door of my house without further incident.

The following morning about 9 a.m. my bedside phone rang.

It was the good doctor calling. "Warren, I'm on my way to church, and I thought that I'd stop by on my way there and remove your catheter. No reason to make you wear it until tomorrow."

Ten minutes later he was at the house. Shortly thereafter, the uncomfortable catheter was removed from my *plumbing fixture.*

I was now free to stand, sit, and move without discomfort. It was a wonderful feeling.

It was even more wonderful to have Dr. B. as my urologist.

No wonder I have thrived so well during my bout with cancer.

Great medical caregivers with a heart. I would certainly number good Dr. B. as a prototype.

For argument's sake we'll say that I was under his care for three months in the interval following radiation. He did his job. He attended to the laundry basket of urinary complaints that I had.

"Before turning you back to Dr. T. I want to discuss something with you that I consider very important. As I see it, you should have no urinary problems for the foreseeable future.

"Warren," he continued. "But, I must warn you that there is no warranty against future problems." He paused. "I have mentioned this to you in the past. Blockage in your urinary tract can crop up any time.

"I would like, to have you equip yourself with a self-catheterization device. Just remember, the farmers that I've told you about. They have been using them for many years. It's a very a simple thing to use. By doing your own self catheterization you can bypass emergency rooms at weird and unexpected hours of day and night."

I'll say no more on the subject. Following his advice I agreed to let him set me up to use the self catheter.

Dr. B. knew of what he spoke. Shortly, thereafter, I found myself using the tube in the morning when I awoke. It was one of those unpleasant chores that I would do a couple times a week. Eventually, I stopped using it. Haven't used the self-help device for more than 18 months. Like a fire extinguisher, at the ready, I have the self-catheter tube in the bathroom awaiting a potential emergency. Like the fire extinguisher I derive no pleasure using it. But if the need should arise I'll be prepared.

*   *   *

It was always a treat to visit Dr. T. Customarily it would be Nurse Te. that would get my show on the road. She would handle the *blood letting* that preceded my *meat and potatoes* visit to the examining room.

After small talk she would take me to the treatment room to await Dr. T.

When he joined me with one of his patented smiles I realized that I was in the right place. When he did his commentary on basketball for the neighboring university I was certain that I was in the right place.

It had been six months since he inserted his digit. It was obvious that he was not out of practice. Talking with his nasal-friendly Jersey accent he wasted little time getting to the point.

"Things with you haven't gotten any better. But not to despair. I am going to send you to one of finest oncologists anywhere. He's the same one that I had sent my mother to.

"His name is Dr. G. He's a young guy, but he's tops. Nobody in his group is any better than him. Matter of fact I'd stack him up against anybody in the business.

I'm going to set you up with an immediate appointment. Believe me, when I tell you, that it's not always so easy to accomplish. But I'm tight with G., and I'm confident that we'll be able to get you into see him real soon."

Chapter 5 *New Ball Game*

My daughter B. came with me for my first visit with Dr. G. He was younger than both of us.

Slender of build - he was a very handsome man.

I was to later learn that his specialties were in Hematology (Blood) and Oncology (Cancer).

Since my daughter had been going through the experience of having a hubby with cancer she was qualified to know the questions that she wanted to ask.

By nature, she takes an aggressive posture of *I want to know what is broken* and *how it's going to be fixed.* As for me, I was inclined to be quite passive. I just felt that Dr. T. would not have referred him to me (with such glowing praise) if Dr. G. was not as promised.

During the visit-meeting he explained that he would be ordering a catscan for me. Then, after studying the results, he and I would again meet. We would then jointly agree upon the treatment that I would be receiving.

It was quite obvious that he had no intention of ram rodding anything down my throat. He wanted me to play a part in determining the course of treatment.

The visit was over. Next, would be the catscan to

be followed by appropriate treatment. My introductory meeting went off smoothly. I liked Dr. G and looked forward to being treated by him.

*   *   *

In a recent conversation with my daughter, she volunteered an observation. Every cancer patient handles the situation differently. Her husband, who is in remission, always trivialized everything that the doctors told him. In my case, she observed, I was totally *out of it* - completely oblivious to whatever the doctors told me.

By way of illustration, she recounted the meeting that I had with the radiation oncologist at which she attended. The meeting, she stated, took place at the hospital that handled my radiation. According to her version, the doctor stated that my cancer had come out of *the envelope*. He further stated that my cancer had reached the Stage 4 level.

If my life were to depend upon it, I can not recall the meeting. To this day, I have no recollection of my daughter ever traveling to the hospital where my radiation took place. By the same token, I have absolutely no recollection of the radiation oncologist's prognosis.

Her husband attests to the fact that he drove us to the hospital that day and that she accompanied me to the meeting with the doctor.

My daughter told me I was "clueless."

Maybe, after all, she is right. It seems possible that I choose to black out any negative information pertaining to my condition. Escapism may be well my way of coping. Who is to say that I'm wrong?

*   *   *

During the first few months of this new medical relationship my personal *plumbing* system required oversight by my *plumber* friend, urologist, Dr. B. Regretfully, I was using the self-catheter system on a regular basis. During the span of one night I even used it three times.

The cause for the disorder was a penile obstruction. Cancerous matter within my penis was blocking the urinary channel.

Both Drs. B&G cooperated fully with regard to my case.

*   *   *

At this juncture it might prove helpful to explain the catscan procedure from my point of view - the patient.

At bedtime on the night prior to the catscan I had to drink a refrigerated bottled drink. Previously, D1 (in Dr. G's office) had issued me two bottles. Laughingly, the drink was called a banana smoothie. In truth, it's a barium sulfate suspension that is flavored with banana. After my bedtime beverage I was prohibited from eating anything until I had completed the catscan.

The second drink had to be consumed the following morning 30 minutes prior to the test. This I did while driving to the hospital for the catscan appointment. It was a 10-minute drive.

At the hospital I checked in at the department's special area. Convinced that my co-pay was in order I took a seat in the waiting area. A technician would come out to summon me.

Five minutes later, a tall young man, J., garbed in hospital greens appeared calling my name.

He lead me down a corridor to a small office where I was directed to a chair. He checked my vital signs and asked a few routine questions.

He then probed my arm for a suitable vein. Simultaneously, he gave me a blow by blow of what was taking place and why.

Upon locating the vein that he wanted he inserted a tube connection (I think it's called a catheter) to the vein. Subsequently, it would be linked to a tube once I got on the catscan machine table. A liquid would then flow into me. According to the tech, I would experience a hot feeling throughout my body. He was right. It was no big deal and only lasted for a few minutes. Most of the procedure took place without the internal body heat condition. Why this was necessary, he did not say - and I didn't ask.

Now, a few details of the procedure from my perspective.

In the center of an average size room is a large table with an donut formed movable contraption on top. (Not a scientific description).

I laid down on my back on the table. The tech connects a tube to the catheter that he had previously inserted in my arm.

I am then reminded that I will experience heat within me and not to be concerned about it. I am then instructed to elevate my two arms.

I am now under the large movable *donut* that will now travel back and forth across my head and upper body. From embedded speakers within the overhead arch I will hear a *monotonous* male *monotone* voice. (I will hear many times).

"Hold your breath."

I do what the voice says. At the same time I have been looking and reading in front and above my range of sight the warning. It is on the arch that surrounds my head and upper body. It reads something like *Do not look into the above beam of light.*

For the umpteenth time I hold my breath until I wonder whether I can hold it a second longer … then the monotonous male voice commands, "Breathe."

That particular sequence is over.

Suddenly, I again hear, "Hold your breath."

Again, just as I feel I have to breathe the voice says, "Breathe."

As I said previously the heated sequence wasn't bad and didn't take too long.

Eventually, the technician returned to me from his control room. He had me alter my position from my back to my side. The order from Dr. G. called for certain specific tests.

The previous process was repeated and included the same droning male voice.

Again, the process stopped. I waited for an eternity (maybe 10 minutes). The films were being reviewed. If the computer screen revealed any distortions, or whatever, the appropriate test would have to be repeated.

At long last, the technician was by my side. "You're all finished. You can get your things and leave when you're ready."

Exactly 10 minutes later I was in the 3rd Floor cafeteria of the hospital. I was eating a breakfast that, any place else, would cost a king's ransom. It cost me $3.25. From the serving line I selected pancakes, corned beef hash, O'Brien potatoes, juice and coffee. Had I selected more prudently it would have been a lot less.

It's little wonder that I saw so many hospital employees eating there with waist lines well beyond the recommended.

Incidentally, people in the know (in my neck of the woods) classify the eatery as the best value within 50 miles (if not more).

It's was a fringe benefit for getting a catscan for me.

I had to wait several days before learning the results of the test from Dr. G.

*　　*　　*

Three days after the catscan I received a call from the oncology clinic. I was told that I had been set up with an appointment to see Dr. G. the following Monday.

At the appointed time, I was in the treatment room with the good doctor. He gave me a quick rundown on the results. If my life depended upon it I could not tell you what the test had revealed.

[COMMENT: I am now of the opinion that at all meetings with the doctor the patient is well advised to bring a notepad. Notes should be taken. As an alternative the patient can bring a companion to do the note taking.]

Having completed his explanation he conducted me to the chemotherapy treatment room. It was here that I underwent more than two hours of chemo. It was my very first treatment.

In a future chapter I will describe my treatments in detail.

*   *   *

A subsequent catscan as reported to me by Dr. G. came over something like this: The cancer has spread from the prostate - coming out of the envelope and going into the liver.

Though, at the time, I knew virtually nothing about the function of the liver I did consider the report very scary. Matter of fact, it scared me so much that I went to the Internet in hopes of coming up with a cure.

Entering the cancer Web site with special attention to liver I performed, what I felt, was a very thorough search. It involved a lot of reading. Each of the options was very technical. In light of the fact that I have never so much as taken a first aid course it seemed foolhardy to tread where seasoned oncologists do. Be that as it may, I did. Like the famed naval quotation *damned the torpedoes full speed ahead* I plowed with both feet into my liver cancer project.

Bingo! A study was being conducted at a large city hospital in a neighboring state. They were looking for individuals with liver cancer for the study.

I did not hesitate to bring this up to Dr. G.'s attention.

He never objected to input by me nor did he ever discourage me from securing outside opinions.

After hearing me out, he looked at me and stated, "But, you don't have liver cancer."

"Oh no," I mumbled. "What kind of cancer do I have?"

"Hormonal Refractory Prostate Cancer," was the good doctor's immediate response.

That incident indicated to me that without some medical training I'm better off not coming up with recommendations as to how I should be treated.

*   *   *

One thing that impresses me so much about Dr. G. is that he always tells it as he believes it is. He is a no-nonsense practitioner.

Early on in our relationship I asked him a very simple question.

"Dr. G., what's my prognosis?"

Spontaneously, he responded with a single word, "Months."

When he looked at me following his answer he must have seen the image of a zombie on my countenance. "I don't mean this month or next month." He said softly.

He never did tell me which month.

Chapter 6   *I Gofer a Twofer*

It all begins as I step through the opened automatic doors.

There have been days when I have felt better. I'm glad that I don't have to look in the mirror to see the reflection of a grumpy old man.

I walk the few steps to the counter, with keys in hand. Before I have the opportunity to turn them over to the ever smiling S. she gives me a very bright and happy smile. She really means it.

"Good morning, Warren. How are you feeling?" It's said with sincerity.

Spontaneously, I feel the frown dissolve and disappear from my face. At that very instant, I feel good. It's the first time since arising some few hours earlier that I have had this great feeling. The very sweet S. has made my day.

I don't even realize it, but she has already taken my keys, isolated the wellness center's plastic scan tag, and registered me. She returns the keys to my hand and throws me a warm smile. She has now turned toward the next patron.

With brisk and determined gait I head for the exercise area.

For me, all is well with the world.

*   *   *

I, like so many others, firmly believe that we should get our money's worth from every expenditure. So, why shouldn't that be the case in matters of health.

It is my goal to work out a minimum of three times a week. I've been following this practice for more than 25 years. Do I do this because I'm an exercise freak? Ans. DEFINITELY NOT. Do I do it because I enjoy it and have nothing better to do? Ans. DEFINITELY NOT.

The reason I exercised in the past and do so now is because I believe that it is good for me.

To validate this theory I would point out, that at 80, I'm still getting up and making an effort to be active.

You might point out (and you could easily be right) that maybe it was genes not exercise that did the trick. To that, I would respond that exercise certainly hasn't done any harm.

In my basement are several pieces of workout equipment.

So, now you might ask if I utilize that equipment at home to its potential. My answer to that is DEFINITELY NOT. Only on those rare occasions when the snow is piled roof high. I might also use it when the roads could be used for ice skating or hockey. At times like that I will use my equipment.

Yes, you're right! And I'll agree with you if you say I'm wasting money. But, hear me out. I am about to explain the formula that I am following. And let me tell you something, "It's working!"

I'm following the *twofer* system. For a very reasonable dues I'm combining a fitness regimen and a social background. For me, it's working. I've stuck to my objective of working out three times a week minimum. On workouts that I miss my whole psyche goes berserk.

AND NOW I'm going to share the magic formula for my success.

For an extended period I have adhered to a scheduled physical fitness regimen. Keep in mind, that I am not an exercise *junkie*. Also remember that I don't exercise because I love it or for the lack of anything better to do. I do it because I BELIEVE that it is good for me.

Like dieters, exercisers must be disciplined. They must maintain a spirit of *go get 'em* on an ongoing basis.

If you know me, you will know that it's not in my nature to be disciplined. In order to achieve the goals that I have outlined it was necessary to have a *crutch*.

Now, the much talked about magic *twofer* formula:

1. I believe that membership in a formal fitness club has helped me accomplish the goal. Said fitness center has the necessary equipment, facilities, and informed personnel to aid me in accomplishing my fitness goals.

2. I believe that most of us are social *animals*. At the fitness center that I attend I have succeeded in bonding with countless individuals. Many of them, I regard as friends. The expectation of seeing many of them on my fitness center visits has proven to be a motivator for me.

CONCLUSION: I am convinced that my life as a cancer victim is thriving better than expected. In great measure I attribute it to my *Socialized Fitness Regimen*

Formula. With it, I am healthier physically and mentally, than I would be without it.

For people with cancer nothing is more important than good physical and mental well being.

*   *   *

MY MEANING OF *Twofer*: Benefit 1 of two benefits for one price. In the case of the fitness center that I attend I pay dues for use of equipment, facilities, and amenities. It also includes the availability of informed and competent personnel.

Before moving on to the second perceived benefit I should give you a quick rundown on my *workout.*

It's duration will vary between 45 minutes to an hour. Generally, I'll kick it off by doing my cycle of some seven or eight machines. I adhere to my current weight and repetition levels. I will then ride a standing bike for 15 minutes.

There are times for, one reason or another, that I will just do the machines or just do the bike for 30 minutes. On my next visit I will do the vice versa. Oft times this deviation will find me back the following day. This will be an extra day, for the week, for me at the center.

Changes such as the above tend to break the monotony of workouts.

Now for Benefit 2 for the same dues. Exposure to the other members while working out. In addition, there is the likelihood that some of them will become social associates at the center. Ultimately some of them will even become friends.

Just think - a physical fitness regimen combined with a social program - all for the same buck.

Let me cite specific examples of how this has worked for me. Hopefully, it will give you a better understanding of the point that I am making.

Without a shadow of a doubt it has contributed to the extension of my life as a cancer victim.

*   *   *

Some three years ago, more or less, I *joined up* for an aerobics class called *Young At Heart*. It was just starting up. It was designed for newcomers to that form of exercise. That classification was designed for me. For more years than I can count I managed to escape the aerobics *animal*.

As I recall, there were only eleven of us - including T., the instructor. My friend G. was the only other male. During the course of our class we were aware of a male face ogling us through the glass part of the room's back door. He appeared to be very interested in what we were doing.

During a water break I snagged on to him and invited him to join us.

The next day GM. became a loyal and faithful member of our group. In his 70s, he's one of the most delightful guys that you could ever find. I was shocked when I learned that he was a close neighbor that I had never met. Our paths, just, had never crossed.

Several years have elapsed.

I no longer belong to that group. Still it thrives bigger than ever before with a regular attendance ranging from 20 to 28 participants. Yes, the *Young At Hearters* continues to thrive with a more elevated level of exercise than at inception.

G. and GM are still tried and true to the cause.
Though no longer aerobicizing with them I, happily,
still continue to maintain a close associationship with
them both.

*   *   *

Then there is SR. Couldn't ask to know a nicer
guy. Everybody seems to know him. He's one of those
happy plain spoken *country boys* with a somewhat acer-
bic tongue-in-cheek manner. For many years he was
the successful operator of his own rural grocery store/
service station combination. Our paths are constantly
crossing while doing the machines or riding the station-
ary bike. I can truthfully say that he is a fun person
that always leaves me upbeat. He's just a good guy that
always leaves you smiling.

It seems that opposites always seem to attract. His
delightful wife, JR, is sweet, calm, unobtrusive, pure of
tongue. She has all the qualities that make for a patient
and loving spouse.

I don't say that SR is the opposite from his wife.
But, whereas he has *never met a stranger* she tends to
operate from a more reserved and private mode.

Guess that's their chemistry for a long and happy
marriage.

*   *   *

I spotted D. heading to the reception desk. From
there he would move to the exit. At the time, I was
working a stomach-crunching machine on the far side of
the machine area. In my pocket was an envelope with a

check covering my veteran's service club dues.

Anything to save 37 cents. I jumped off the tummy cruncher and ran after him. He was well ahead of me. He has a hearing problem and could not hear me shouting his name. I had deserted my machine and was at his heels as he exited the facility.

Slender and well proportioned D. was in early to mid-60s. He still moved at his customary brisk military gait. I did catch up with him and handed him the envelope.

After thanking me, he then surprised me by asking, "Do you mind if I ask you a personal question?"

I've known D. for about five years. First met him at church. Subsequently, I connected with him through his executive connection with a local veteran organization. We also see each other at the fitness center on a very regular basis.

A retired regular army officer with a distinguished career he and his wife J. have come to this area to enjoy their retirement.

"Of course," was my immediate response to his halting question.

"May I ask, what kind of cancer do you have?" Asked with trepidation.

"Prostate cancer," was my immediate answer.

He then explained that he had just gone to his PCP, an internist, for his annual physical. In the course of the exam the doctor mentioned that it had been a long time since he had been given a chest X-ray.

The subsequent X-ray disclosed a suspicious area on the lung. Further study confirmed that the performance of a biopsy would be the next prudent step.

After sharing that report with me, he observed. "But, what's really worrying me is that J. (his wife) has a suspicious spot on her pancreas." He then paused for a few seconds before adding, "there's a history of pancreatic cancer in her immediate family."

Socialization at the wellness center takes many forms. Life just goes on.

The good news for this lovely couple is that they are fortunate in having physicians that have probed into all facets of their health and background. D: Insisting that he submit to an X-ray. J: Awareness of family history and following through.

Though, there are never guarantees in cancer or, for that matter, with life, the following is a given: The earlier a cancer problem is caught the better it is for cure.

In both instances the saying to be *forewarned is to be forearmed.* In the meantime *the jury is out on both D&J.* Hopefully, their trip will be an easy one.

Oft times people are heard to observe about situations such as theirs by uttering, "It just isn't fair."

In response I would respond with the French phrase *c'est la vie.* (That's life.)

*   *   *

Then there is J. whom I have known for many years. He is a retired educator who had elevated to the higher strata of local school administration.

He is to be admired for his verve for life and the community. Though a recovered heart patient with a very serious history he moves at full pace. His competitive juices now flow to tennis. In his younger day he was a pretty fair to middlin' pitcher in local adult baseball leagues.

J. has never been known to hide his opinion on any facet of life. He serves on governmental commissions and boards too numerous to mention. Constantly, he publicly expresses his opinion on timely subjects as they come to the public forefront.

In addition to his faithful use of the wellness center's tennis courts he is sure to keep the fitness machines busy. He even finds time to serve the center as a member of their advisory board.

Not a day goes by that he doesn't corner me and volunteer some interesting tidbit of either info or opinion. All the while, he encourages me to continue to fight the good battle. I consider this very rugged individualist a wonderful friend that I can always count upon.

*   *   *

Then there is B., the retired pharmacy owner, that I had always dealt with in years gone by. Unlike J (above) B. is mild mannered and very reserved. This does not mean that he is without opinion. He's a very well informed individual and knowledgeable on so much. He's just a very private-type person.

For years he had attended to his cancer-afflicted wife. She died several years ago. It has been a very difficult loss for him.

I can recall admiring his gumption as he daily walked his set course covering the downtown streets of our town. This solitary form of exercise had served as his principal means of conditioning.

I was so happy to see him frequenting the wellness center where he regularly adheres to a regimen of fitness. He does the machine thing along with mixing with his fellow members. Our paths often cross giving us the opportunity to make small talk.

It's good to know that B. is there for me. Hopefully, he knows that I, too, am there for him.

* * *

Then there is young M., the son of a retired physician and lovely wife. Young M. is an avid work-outer. He loves people and will always go out of his way to greet me and inquire about me. He is a wonderful and very special young man.

* * *

For more than 25 years I had been a regular attending member of a weekly meeting service club. Said group met in a neighboring community to that of my residence. After my diagnosis, I felt it necessary to drop my membership. It had been a very happy run and I regretted, so very much, the need to sever my ties with the club and its members.

What has been so wonderful about the wellness center is the fact that it serves both my community and the neighboring one of which the club is located. In the course of doing *my thing* I have run into at least a half-dozen members of the club.

* * *

The Table - Being a creature of habit I generally complete my regimen of *self-induced torture* (Just Joking!!!) between 11:00 and 11:10 each morning. It is then, with towel in hand, I depart the machine and weights area. I take the short walk to the newly opened cafe in the adjoining newly constructed building.

In the cafe are some half-dozen circular tables surrounded by chairs. At the particular time that I arrive most of the tables are usually empty. I choose a vacant one and toss my towel atop a chair. Thence, I proceed to the coffee machine in the other part of the cafe.

By the time that I return with my filled cup the first of my regular tablemates appears. It's GS, a tall, slender guy ever armed with an overflowing repertoire of jokes. I'd peg him at either the tail end of his 50s or early part of his 60s. His worldwide service as a cook in the U.S. Army came to a premature end because of health and subsequent medical discharge.

Industriously, he went the way of the *double dipper*. For some 13 years he served as a cook at a state correction institution in the neighboring community. His era of *double dipping* recently came to an inglorious end when the state unceremoniously condemned the institution.

GS, if anybody, has to be the anchor person for our *table*. Never at a loss for words, there are always stories to recount or jokes to tell. Aside from his own physical health, his biggest concern was expressed by his recent question to our group: "Why is the Statue of Liberty considered part of New York state when it lays within the boundaries of New Jersey?" It is obvious from where he originally hails.

He's extremely generous and never hesitates to speak with his purse if one of us should be experiencing a temporary financial shortfall at the cafe.

In no more than days after meeting, he and I had established a very close bond. Intuitively, I feel that I can always count upon him if the need should arise.

This had vividly come to pass a week ago. I was in the process of leaving the wellness center - he was just arriving. He explained that he was arriving late because of some necessary errands - "I had to go to W to buy some cat food."

I responded, "I've got to stop by the doctor's office. My red count was real low, and I'm afraid that I'm going to have another blood transfusion." (NOTE: Because of extremely low red blood count - anemia.)

His expression became very concerned, "You need blood - you've got it."

I assured him that I did not.

GS is truly one in a million.

*   *   *

GS and myself had been chatting between sips of coffee for several minutes when D & S enter the cafe area. They are regulars at the table.

They greet us both with giant smiles. After dropping their personal effects on the table they prepare to proceed to the coffee machine. Before leaving D. looks at our cups, "Either of you guys need some more?"

We thank the pretty blonde and assure her that we are in *good shape.*

D.'s in her 30s, a married homemaker, with a child that attends elementary school. She has a perpetual smile that goes along with her cheerful good nature. She is always solicitous of my condition. She never fails to ask how she can be of service to me.

Just the other day the mail carrier left a Halloween card in my mailbox from her. Believe me when I tell you that this one had all of the *bangles and bows.*

Without a doubt it was one of the flashiest cards I have ever received. For just an instant I contemplated upon it and wondered if it would light up like a neon sign. On its back cover she had inscribed the notation that it was coming from one of the people at the *table*.

People like D. give me one more reason to smile and one less reason to frown.

By her side was the low keyed S., a very pleasant gal with hubby and high school attending son. She tended to have a few extra pounds more than she really wanted to carry. She conceded that she had not yet tackled that problem in the fashion that she really wanted.

She has beautiful black hair and appears to be in her early 40s. S. is earnest and caring with a soft spoken manner - she's an integral and ideal occupant of the table.

Next to arrive is K. She's slight of build and very pretty. I now realize that she has to be in her early 40s.

Listen to how I had originally miscalculated her age upon first meeting her.

I had promised to get her a copy of my latest murder mystery, *Marvelous Maggie*, (might as well get in a plug). I made the drive to her home. Upon arrival, I noted her handsome hubby navigating his small tractor. It was doing what small tractors do on the land surrounding their home. (Don't forget that I come from the city.)

K. was scurrying about among the pretty flowers presumably doing things with said flowers. She was wearing work gloves and holding a garden tool. Standing nearby was a very attractive girl that I guessed to be either 16 or 17 (at most). By now I had just been introduced to her by K. at the same time that she introduced hubby, D.

Book in hand, and the two elders otherwise occupied, I handed the book to their daughter. Jokingly, I added, "Make sure you hand it over to the folks without reading it. I'm just a wee bit afraid that it's a bit too spicy." I then added, with a smile. "It's R-rated for gals your age."

K. grinned. "Don't worry, Warren, she's 21 and visiting us from college in Charleston."

Like mother like daughter, they both looked younger than their years. It was then that I changed my original guess of K.'s age from 30s to 40s. It was a sure bet that she hadn't conceived at nine years of age.

K. is a very talented individual with a natural bent for writing.

After reading my book she sent me a glowing tribute in which she detailed all the reasons that she so thoroughly enjoyed the book.

As I read her review (which I very much wish had also been elicited from the reviewer at *The New York Times*) I thought to myself: "If only I had the ability to express myself as does K."

I've received from her both e-mail and the conventional kind. I am inspired to continue with my work. She also motivates me to continue fighting my physical battles.

Yes, K. has caused my creative juices to boil by her encouragement. At the same time it makes me focus on things other than me.

For me, K. serves as a wonderful weapon against the scourge of the Big "C."

*   *   *

Next to the *table* is my old "Bud" G. He stakes out a chair and then heads back to the coffee. Upon returning, he seats himself across the table from me. He offers a smile and commences to sip from the Styrofoam cup. During the 20 minutes that he is there I doubt that he says more than a couple dozen words.

He is exceedingly admired by the others from the group.

*   *   *

The next to pass through the entryway is the distinguished looking GM. He, drags a chair over from an adjoining table and joins us. He will not be drinking coffee. He awaits his wife, F., to complete her workout. Then they will be going to the hospital cafeteria for their lunch.

An old-timer to the community GM is a wealth of information on the yesteryear of the area. He's got an excellent sense of humor. It's an entirely different brand from that of the man from Jersey. He's a very well-liked individual.

Incidentally, he and F. are the parents of the good Nurse Te. in Dr. T.'s office.

*   *   *

Like an object being propelled by a tropical wind comes the next individual through the portals. He's wearing his hallmark workout outfit of a dark undershirt that can easily pass as a T-shirt. He's also wearing dark workout shorts.

It's the radiant SR whose path I cross on virtually each and every workout date.

Upon spotting me, he descends upon me from the

rear. He leans over so he can whisper into my ear some mild obscenity. Then, with a smile he scurries to another table for a chair. He has now joined the *table*.

He only remains a few minutes - long enough to inject a new spirit of humor to the proceedings. He departs as quickly as he arrived.

He is so very real and so very likeable. Though, he's never so indicated I have absolutely no doubt that I can count upon him in time of need.

*   *   *

Wearing a T-shirt emblazoned with U.S. Marines is E.

A newcomer to the *table* - he's very outgoing and fits in well with the group. In his past life he was a design engineer. Though we have not known him long we have ascertained one thing: He totally disagrees with GS's position on Lady Liberty's native state. E.'s position is that *The Lady* is a duly recognized resident of the "Empire State." Note: Whereas E. is from NY it should be noted that GS is from the Garden State of NJ.

E. like GS is endowed with a large repertoire of jokes. As a man of humor he actively contributes to the overboisterousness that frequently erupts from the *table*.

Incidentally, today E. and I., actively debated the U.S. foreign policy stand. It was heated and went back to WWI. At one point it even drifted back to the era of James Monroe. I leaned slightly to the position espoused by the long dead president while E. defended the current one.

We quit on the note that politics was always king. Neither of us would deny that various ethnic and national lobbying groups influenced the course of our nation's foreign policy. We now had a peaceful resolution to the debate.

During the discussion we had the *table* to ourselves.

*   *   *

There is nothing extra special or unusual about the *table*. It's just a group of guys and gals that try to get together for a few minutes each day at the wellness center during the course of the workout day.

Nothing said is earth shaking or for the ages.

So, what's the big deal?, you might ask.

There is no big deal, I would respond.

I can only tell you this. (1) I look forward to being with them. (2) I enjoy their company collectively or individually. (3) It's one more reason for me to fulfill my exercise commitment on a given day.

And last but far from least: After leaving them I feel better mentally. That makes me feel better physically.

Combine the both and I'll tell you this: As a cancer patient I've had another great day.

*   *   *

Always the one with an eye that takes it all in, I can not forget the pretty T. She was the trainer that led our *Young at Heart* aerobics group beginning with Day 1. From 11 beginners to more than three times that number she has cultivated some very competent aerobicists.

Way back when - I was in the group she displayed all of the qualities of a saint in getting me started. From her personal interest in converting me from bumble head to acceptable she did a yeoman job. I shall never forget.

To the present she still inquires from mutual acquaintances about me. On those occasions that we pass each other it's always an occasion that I treasure.

*   *   *

With that same observant eye I think of the very pretty and athletic Dr. D., the dentist. Our paths first crossed at a previous fitness center that we both attended. We have been friends ever since.

Since my diagnosis she has ever been mindful of my needs. I can remember the occasion more than a year ago when I was on a carrot juice kick. The particular label that I used was only obtainable at a store in a nearby town. Imagine my surprise to find a case of same that she purchased. She dropped it off at my front door. She bought it for me out of the goodness of her heart.

She's a very special person that would do anything for me should the situation dictate.

With friends like T. and Dr. D. I'm glad that this geriatric cancer victim has an observing eye.

Chapter 7   *The Chemo Factory*

You will recall that my cancer treatment commenced with radiation involving 60-mile round trips daily.

Had the above been successful it would not have been necessary to write this chapter. But, as I like to say, *c'est la vie.*

For the greater part of the past two years I have been making one trip a week for my chemotherapy treatment. Instead of a 30-mile journey I only go four.

The cancer center occupies a modern one-story brick building with convenient parking in front. It's a beautiful rural area that adjoins the modern regional medical center that serves the adjacent communities. Incidentally, it's no more than a two-minute drive to the wellness center. My PCP, urologist, and orthopedist are in a building that adjoins the hospital. (Like an old car it takes a lot of repair people for an old man).

It's an area that abounds with medical facilities surrounded by rolling hills and green grass fields. An interstate and convenient state roads reach here from the neighboring communities.

Each Monday I customarily drive to the parking area in front of the cancer center. From there it's a hop, skip, and a jump (figurative) to the entrance of the building. I go through it. Once inside, I hang my jacket on the rack located in the hallway. One more door, and I'm in the waiting room. There are several waiting patients spotted throughout the room.

I check in with C., the pretty *traffic cop*, who efficiently keeps the flow of traffic moving from her station. She is seated behind the sliding glass window with computer and phone by her fingers. She's in a large office crammed with patient files. Customarily, there are two or three other young ladies back there.

One of them is O. who's responsible for insurance and the red tape that goes with it. At the moment she's busy banging away at her PC.

The other young lady is D1. She's a human spark plug - she's a human dynamo. I will visit her on the way out. She, too, is located behind a sliding glass window. Her's is on the other side of the door that separates the waiting room from the rest of the facility.

I have taken one of the empty chairs located near the *traffic cop* and patiently await my turn to be called.

I'm summoned after a wait of about 10 minutes. C. slides her window open and instructs me to go back.

I push the glass-topped door. If I turn left I'm at the special nursing station manned by Nurse J. She does the prelim work on patients that will be making a doctor's visit. From her station a short hallway leads to the private treatment rooms and doctors' offices.

Close by is the lab where blood and other specimens are tested. The nursing staff take samples from virtually every patient on every visit.

On this day I follow the corridor that leads to what I have tagged the *Chemo Pavilion.*

Having reached the chemo area, I momentarily close my eyes and envision myself entering the cocktail lounge of a superliner. I see a semi-circular layout lined with windows from which one can see the peaceful water. I imagine that I'm on a cruise ship. I can envision an inviting lounge looking out upon the sea. I open my eyes and realize that I'm not on the ship's upper deck.

I am now gazing through the semi-circle bank of windows at the far end of the *chemo pavilion*. I look out on the verdant hills of the scenic Shenandoah Valley not the blue waters of the Caribbean.

Back to reality! Forward of the windows, following the same semi-circular path are five patient occupied *Lazy Boy* recliners. To the side of each chair stands an IV pole with hanging and working plastic bags.

Facing the window shielding patients, some six feet distant, and following the same parallel path are four more patients upon recliners.

Off to the side is the large nurse's station from which the three nurses on duty operate. (Not the scalpel variety). Adjacent to the station is the room from which they mix the prescribed chemo formulas.

On the corridor that I have just walked are two restrooms easily accessible to the patients. Since the IV poles are on wheels it's just a matter of walking and wheeling the pole alongside.

There is a magazine rack - for the most part, it is used by patient accompanists. Patients, for some reason or other, have an aversion to reading old magazines.

Within eyeshot of the patients is a snack area complete with a mini fridge. Soft drinks, juices, and specialties such as Ensure and Boost are within. For eating pleasure there is a supply of chips, peanut butter crackers, Doritos items, Lays items, and other quick fixes. The snacks have a propensity for making one thirsty.

Upon entering the chemo area, to one's left, is a corridor that leads to the doctor's offices and treatment rooms.

Working today is Nurse S., very knowledgeable and equally very no-nonsense. She is caring - an attribute that I recognize in the other two.

Then there is Nurse D2, a tall and slender brunette. She, too, is very caring and competent. She and I have established a special kind of relationship. It is one in which I flagrantly delight in teasing her in front of others. I follow the theme that she "loses points" every time she hurts me. This would take place in the course of giving me shots, taking my blood, or searching for a vein. Happily for me, being a good sport is one of her attributes.

[NOTE: I am at this instant doing an edit of this page. Just yesterday while submitting to a blood test a fellow patient observed me. "If you relaxed your arm you would not feel any pain or discomfort." I realized that she was right. You see, one is never too old to learn.]

Then, relatively new to the roster is Nurse B. Though I do not know her as well as the others this mild-mannered nurse appears to be very caring and knowl-edgeable.

Even newer to the staff (Day 1 - today), fresh from the shops of Bal Harbor in Miami Beach, Florida, comes Nurse Da.

NOTE: Nurse Da took some blood from me that precipitated the suggestion in the preceding NOTE.

The nursing staff is rounded out by two nurse practitioners.

Heading up the operation are four oncologists, one of them being my own Dr. G.

On rare occasion it has been necessary to be attended by one of the others. I have absolutely no qualms about any of the other two men or one woman. They all know their *stuff.*

This cancer center is a satellite operation for the group. Their main operation is located in a private hospital in a city 25 miles from my home. They also operate another satellite operation in another community.

Their operation functions on the scheduling of a single physician to my facility on a specified day of the week. As you have already been told, Dr. G. is a Monday person.

It is now departure time for me.

Before exiting the threshold leading to the waiting room I pass the energetic dynamo, herself - the *gatekeeper*, D1. In addition to being responsible for all scheduling she has her fingers on a host of other things.

Scheduling at an oncology facility is a major league headache for those administering the function. Regimens are forever being changed creating scheduling problems. Emergencies, needless to say, create more problems. All of these things coupled with already existing patient care loads at a given time fit into the mix.

There is little doubt that the qualities of a magician make for a good gatekeeper.

Chapter 8   *All the Artillery*

All my travails began in October 2000. It was in October 2001 that I entered into the next major battle in my personal war against the *Big C* - cancer.

When it was first announced to me that I had been diagnosed with cancer it was as if I had been told that my life had come to an end. Deep within me my emotions became very confused. First of all, I was ashamed - embarrassed, if you will. I did not want others to know. I wanted to keep it a secret.

It did not take long for me to adjust my sights - so to speak. I did the radiation thing.

Had it done the job I would not be here. In chapter 7, I walked you through the *palace* in which I have been coming since October 2001.

It is my hope to give you an overview of what I have encountered since that date. Though I talk and deal with things medical I must, once again, remind you that I know nothing medical. All that I will tell you is what treatment I received according to my noteless recollections. I have not even researched my chart.

My purpose is to make this readily understandable

to any layperson: patient or caregiver. It's from the perspective of ONE cancer patient - ME.

I also caution you to remember that the sequence of treatments that I speak about may not be in proper order. In any event the gist of the tale will not be compromised.

For almost two years I received, on a quarterly basis, an injection into the hip called Lupron. As I understand it, the active hormones are very much to the liking of the cancer cells. The more active they become the more active becomes the cancer.

The Lupron, as I understand it, caused my hormones to be pushed to the background. This would cause the cancer cells to go back in hiding from a very active environment. Net result to me would be a less active cancer.

Were there any side effects? Yes, is my unequivocal response. The one that I recall the most was *hot flashes*. I could *hear* my saintly wife, Kay, looking down at me. She would be pointing her finger toward me and with a knowing smirk utter, "And now you know, Mr. Smartie, what I had been telling you ..."

A second side effect - and a rather strange one - was an enlargement of my breasts.

If only through osmosis I could have given said effect to some needy individual.

Lupron was given in addition to chemotherapy.

Another treatment that I received was Thalidomide. You may recall the rash of deformed babies that were born some years back. It was contended that the mothers had, previous to conception, ingested this drug.

I can not recall how long I took the drug or whether there were any side effects. On the other hand I do recall calling the pharmaceutical manufacturer and submitting to an oral examination. I do recall that I passed the quiz.

Some of the questions were: Have you had any unprotected sex and did I intend to have any? Did I plan on siring any children while taking this drug? There were other questions that I can not recall. Obviously, I gave them the answers they wanted to hear. Frankly, I was quite amused -flattered would be better. After all, I was around 79 at the time.

CHEMOTHERAPY - The use of chemical agents in the treatment or control of disease.

From the definition you can readily see that this form of treatment can be administered with unlimited possibilities. I point this out so that you will realize that each patient is administered a specific formula of drugs. The attending physician attempts to prescribe the formulation that he/she feels can best do the job for the specific case.

For me it was a formulation in which Taxol was the dominant chemical.

Occupying one of the recliners - my Monday morning agenda was about to commence. Nurse D2 started it by rolling her little table in front of me.

Though I never thought of calling this gorgeous *thing* Dracula she commenced her activity by pricking my finger with what I liked calling a stapling machine. She removed a blood sample.

Upon completion, she scurried to the lab.

[If my education from ER (the TV program) is good D2 has done a CBC (complete blood count).

On this next point I'm reasonably certain of which I speak. Our blood consists of three main components: red cells, white cells, and platelets. All three are continuously being manufactured by our bone marrow.

The chemo procedure can cause our cell count to go down. It is for that reason that it is constantly monitored prior to treatment. It is also performed on a regular basis between treatments.

Red count controls the energy. Let it get too low and you contract anemia. Note: I can speak from experience. On two occasions I required blood transfusions.

White cells control the immune system. Let it fall too low and the patient becomes unduly exposed to infection.

The platelets help to curb the bleeding by stopping up the blood vessel leaks.

Some minutes later D2 returns advising me that my red count is low. My white count and platelets are OK.

Fortunately, my red count fell within acceptable parameters. Therefore, I am able to receive chemo. Had I fallen much lower on red count they would have *held* me back, that day, from treatment.

Nurse D2, once again, disappeared. This time she went to the room adjacent to the nurses' station where she prepared the formulation for my regimen.

Some five minutes later she returned carrying several plastic bags filled with clear solutions.

She hung the bags on the IV pole. Then she began "excavating" for a vein in my arm. Once she found what she was seeking she inserted the little catheter which was then connected to the delivery tube attached to the first plastic IV bag. She would always start off with a bagful of anti-nausea drug.

Though the infusion of this drug took quite a long time to complete I NEVER objected. I'm not one for nausea - and, happily over two years, I have not suffered an attack as the result of chemo.

This was followed up with a bag of the Taxol. Whether there was a third bag containing saline solution I can not say. Suffice to say, the entire process took a bit more than two hours.

You might wonder if there was pain involved in the process and the answer would be no.

Incidentally, before I left the session Nurse D2 administered a shot of Procrit into my arm. The purpose was to help elevate my red count.

What would I do during the time that I was receiving the chemo?

(a) I would make a trip to the *john.*

(b) I might read the *paper* that I brought with me.

(c) I might bring a book or a magazine.

(d) I might work on a writing project in progress.

(e) I would make a trip to the *john.*

(f) I might chat with a near-by comrade that I knew. (Over time you get to know many)

(g) I might go over to the snack bar for refreshments.

(h) On rare occasions I might snooze.

(i) I'd stare at the bag atop the IV pole to see if it was coming close to being empty. *A watched pot never boils.*

At long last, I might ring the bell by my side (if it was staff lunch hour) to let them know the bag was empty. OR more times than not, either D2 or one of the other nurses would either disconnect me or hook me up to the next bag of the regimen. In any event, after some two hours I was usually disconnected.

General Side Effects From Any and All Regimens that I underwent.

From *the get go* let me state, unequivocally, that no two patients get the same side effects from any given regimen. In my case, I can recall some very pronounced ones.

(1) Numbness in my feet (I believe that they refer to this as neuropathy). It's a strange malady. One day during warm weather I walked out to the street newspaper tube and happened to look down. Would you believe that I was just wearing one sandal? Never even knew it.

(2) Loss of feeling and sensitivity in my fingers and hands. Brittle nails. Have even lost large sections of individual toe nails. Loss of strength in hands causing difficulty in performing routine functions with hands (such as opening things that you buy at the supermarket.

(3) GI system gets all screwed up going from one extreme to another.

(4) GU system: Note: Whether this is side effect or product of disease or just the aging process???? Edema. Extreme water retention creating need for diuretics and the wearing of long hose. I had to constantly lubricate the affected legs. By-product: Spend most of the time, day or night, in *john*.

(5) Loss of hair on scalp. Good News: Young women that have ignored me in the past came over to admiringly pat my head. "Why do you wait until I'm bald before you pay attention to me?" I would ask.

Their universal response, "Because bald is sexy!"

More good news: Instead of shaving daily I don't shave at all.

(6) Taste Buds. Some times there can be a loss of appetite. Sometimes items of food that, at one time, you liked, you no longer enjoy. Conversely, things that you didn't like you now enjoy. Some times you just don't

know. Some times your appetite becomes a problem. Fortunately for me I am now eating quite well. My weight, from water reduction, has gone down from 180 pounds to 150 pounds. Waistline from 40" to 37." My eating habits are unreal. I eat sufficiently at each meal but portions are moderate. Two hours after eating a meal I am snacking. My question: Why could I not weigh and eat as I do now, when I was younger?

(7) Mouth lesions and other minor throat disorders. Generally, through repeated warm salt water gargles this condition will disappear.

(8) Balance problems: Equilibrium is a constant concern. Am now trying exercises involving standing behind chair and moving each leg with *reps* in designated directions. Have problems ascending and descending steps. Special problems at stadium when attending sporting events. Decidedly difficult standing up after an extended period of time sitting.

(9) Problems elevating from sitting to standing position - must use hands and arms to push up. Unable to depend on legs by themselves to rise. Am now trying exercise which involves repeatedly standing from sitting position with use of hands.

(10) Periods in which I suffer from fatigue - sometimes extreme. They tell you to keep as active during these episodes and not give in to it. Weekly shot of Procrit helps to improve the disorder. For me, it has not been too long lasting.

(11) Glazing over eyes - feels like there is a film that causes blurry vision. In my own specific case I have lost my eyelashes on my left eye. This has created some minor problems. My ophthalmologist Dr. G. has prescribed a dry eyes prescription. Incidentally, he has also

treated me for an infected right eye and prescribed antibiotic drops. Subsequently, the left eye became infected.

(12) Edema connection. I have already commented
that this condition may not be a side effect. On the other
hand, I have on, two occasions, undergone *angry* redden-
ing of my affected leg(s) along with leaking spots. This is
a serious concern. The danger of cellulitis is very likely.
Treatment has been antibiotics for a period of 10 days.

Do not forget that the white count controls immune
system. Infections are easy to come by and hard to heal.

On two occasions I was ordered to have blood
transfusions. The first time I required three units and
required an overnight stay at the hospital. The second
time I required two units. On this, I was treated as an
outpatient. This was for Anemia.

As I recall, the three-unit procedure took 12 hours
and the two-unit transfusion ran about eight hours. In
both cases the procedures were painless. I could even
watch the provided TV or read.

*   *   *

Following my round of Taxol chemo I moved to
another regimen. Good Dr. G. was aware of my complaints. They were about the extreme numbness of
my feet (neuropathy) and the overwhelming sensitivity
problems in my hands.

The doc is not the kind of guy that wants to see
his patients suffer. Upon hearing my story he opted to
adjust my chemo regimen. He switched me from the
Taxol to a derivative of it called Taxotere.

If memory serves me, on the day prior to chemo I
had to take 70 calcitriol pills.

I recall, at a meeting of the local prostate cancer support group speaking with the lecturing physician. He was an authority on prostate cancer. I complained about having to take so many pills. He responded by telling me that I should have been happy that I didn't weigh 300 pounds. Had I weighed that much it would have been necessary for me to take 240 pills in a day.

*   *   *

Why don't we take a *time out* from the story of my chemo to inject an unexpected complication (not basketball tickets).

The incident took place on the morning after my course of chemo. I awoke with a slight pain in the chest region. It had prevailed slightly on the two previous days. It had been mild and barely noticeable. On the morning in question it felt more pronounced. It was located high in the chest region and quite deep.

As I got out of bed I was overcome by nausea. (Nurse S. had always instructed me to call *day or night* if ever I had fever.)

By my bed I have a phone with a portable receiver. I called the cancer center and spoke with Nurse S. I complained about my nausea … in the midst of a sentence I double timed to the commode and commenced *barfing*.

I've never lived it down from Nurse S. Can you imagine? I had carried the portable phone with me. She could hear the entire episode taking place. (And without commercial interruptions, to boot).

When I had completed the vomit process she asked me if I had a fever.

"No, I really don't think so."

"Well, if you should, you get yourself in here pronto," were her final words.

I returned to my bed. Before getting back under the covers I opened the drawer to the bedside table. From it I removed the digital thermometer that had been given to me at the cancer clinic. On the hard plastic case was the word Neupogen (R). Removing the thermometer and placing it in my mouth revealed a new truth (for me). I now realized that I didn't know everything. My temp was 101.

Post haste I went to the cancer place and the good Nurse S.

Within the hour, I found myself in my own bed in my own private room of the nearby medical center.

I had been diagnosed with a blood clot in my lung.

I was treated for same and discharged a day or so later. Since that time I have been taking, what I laughingly refer to, as *rat poison*. Officially the drug is called Coumadin. It's an anticoagulant (blood thinner). Currently, I take 5 mg. a day.

Happily, since that episode several years ago there has been no recurrence of the problem.

Once again, I must observe that I have no way of knowing whether the blood clot was in any way associated with the cancer or the treatment. I can only report that it took place during my *cancerwatch*.

*   *   *

Recently, I complained about a slight nagging pain. It felt to me as if it was muscular. As I recall, it prevailed in the region under and behind my shoulder. Dr.

G., always one for touching *all the bases*, dispatched me to the hospital for a bonescan.

The results, though inconclusive, indicated that there had been signs of a bruise in the area of complaint. Happily, the discomfort subsequently disappeared and the bone business has been put to rest.

*   *   *

Some months ago I could have used an appointment book exclusively for my daily meds schedule. I was taking pills for: blood pressure, cholesterol, bladder problems, arthritis. In addition I was taking a slew of vitamins. As you can see, the intake of all these wonderful pellets was designed to give me a long and healthy life.

Combine the above, with the high powered cancer medication being infused and ingested and something had to give.

Like the explosion of Mount Vesuvius so, too, my system, blew sky high one morning. My body had broken out from top to bottom.

A quick trip to my ever working Dr. G. resulted in an immediate decision. "Cut out everything that you are taking … everything!"

Needless to say, the anti-cancer chemo process continued without detour.

You might be interested on how I have fared, one year later, without the benefit of the discontinued medication.

Blood Pressure: It has never been so normal in my entire life. Cholesterol: I don't have the vaguest. Just know that I passed 80 and I'm eating well and am still functioning without problem. Bladder: Seems to be carrying its load. Arthritis: The problem with my hand is resolved with wrist braces. Not a perfect solution but one that is adequate. Vitamins: I seem to be thriving just as well.

Immediately following the episode I opted to visit my friend Dr. P., dermatologist. Some years earlier while attending a baseball game I contracted a *major-league breakout* of my face. It was then that he diagnosed it as an allergic reaction to the drug that I was taking. Evidently direct sunlight and the drug did not make for a happy combination. He gave me a steroid, and my problem was resolved.

Since my breakout this time was even more extensive and more uncomfortable I felt that it might be in my best interests to call upon his services.

Once again, he went the steroid route but it was not the quick fix of my previous problem.

And besides - there was a complication this time; namely, Edema.

I had a pretty nasty case of the above. Whether it had anything to do with my cancer or the treatment I can not say. None of my doctors would or could say how it was caused. Suffice to say I had it.

As I write this, it has been more than a year that I have been fighting it.

What is it? Without getting technical I would just say that the system retains too much fluid. This overflow seems to form a *reservoir* in my legs and feet. The feet balloon up and the lower part of the legs swell and become an angry red. No question about it but it is uncomfortable and definitely impedes one's ability to walk. The condition if allowed to go unchecked can result in a quick trip to the hospital for the treatment of cellulitis.

Gravity carrying the fluid to the legs can pose a problem. The fluid wants to escape through pores in the legs. Little blisters open up on the leg and the fluid oozes out. Concurrently, the bacteria from the outside can come back in through those same opened lesions. Not good!

When Dr. P. was treating me for my drug interaction problem he was working with a *double-edged sword,* so to speak. The ingestion of the steroid definitely addressed the problem for the drug interaction. At the same time it acted as a detriment to the Edema. Evidently, the steroid impeded the efficient discharge of fluid from my system.

In a matter of weeks the problem from the drug reaction was healed. It was then that I decided that I would continue with my friend Dr. P. for treatment.

I did not tell you that while all this was going on I was being attended by a podiatrist.

Unfortunately, the old saying that *too many cooks spoil the broth* applied. The podiatrist was advocating a surgical solution to an ulcer that had formed within one of my toes. My oncologist was opposed to that option.

Since it was also a dermatological problem I decided that I would let Dr. P. work on that along with his other assignments

Now, back to the specific problem of Edema.

One definite side effect of chemo is the fact that it will kill the good healthy cells along with the bad cancer cells. Unfortunately, some of the good ones could have been present to help cure the Edema. Without those healthy cells being available the Edema cure moves in low gear.

What is the cause for the Edema? Who knows?

Maybe the cancer. Maybe not. Maybe a side effect of the chemo and maybe not. In all probability, it is unrelated to the two that I have just mentioned. I think that it is more likely that I would have just gotten it from fair *wear and tear* even if I had never contracted cancer.

MY CONCLUSION: What I do know is that the chemo treatment indiscriminately kills healthy cells in the body as well as the cancer cells. Some of the healthy ones could have taken care of the Edema. Some of those cells could have also fought infections that seem to frequently crop up. So, I guess, one could say that a connection exists between some of my non-cancer-related maladies with the cancer treatment, itself.

Dr. P., in cooperation with the oncologist, has placed me on a diuretic, Lasix. I started with 40 mg. Suffice to say, I take the tablet before getting out of bed. For the next two to three hours I'm running to the *john* with extreme urgency on a very regular basis.

In addition, he had me wearing support hose. Happily, he has relented somewhat. He now permits me to wear conventional knee-high hose or tube stockings. It's more comfortable than the compressed hosiery.

During recent months my Edema has gotten angrier. My erstwhile friend, Dr. P. has increased my dosage of Lasix to 60 mg. This entails longer frequency of round trips to the *john*.

As I write this I must report that last week Dr. P. suspected that I was becoming a candidate for cellulitis. I was then, for the next 10 days, ordered to take four antibiotic capsules a day. In addition, I was to take 60 mg. of Lasix each day. He also insisted that I keep my legs and feet lubricated with a Vaseline-type gel. At the time of his diagnosis my legs bothered me along with my mobility being impaired. I have had better days.

The condition cleared up for a period of about 10 days.

It has returned along with an eye infection.

I have resumed with the same course of antibiotics for the edema. Concurrently, I am using the same antibiotic eye drops for my left eye that I had recently used on my right eye.

NOTE: I will see the dermatologist tomorrow and the ophthalmologist the day after tomorrow.

NOTE AGAIN: If you are not a hypochondriac before the diagnosis you certainly become one after diagnosis. (Ha! Ha!)

Following the initial course of antibiotics for the Edema everything returned to normal, and I felt great. Ditto with my right eye.

With the help of doctors, drugs, and prayers the same will soon occur.

Blue skies always follow storms.

One final thought about swollen feet and Edema.

Recalling my days in the infantry I can honestly say that I fully appreciate the importance of *happy feet.*

*   *   *

You may wonder why I have devoted so much time to the discussion of my diverse non-cancer related ailments.

My answer to you is very clear. Cancer patients not only deal with their cancer but also the full mix of maladies that hit non-cancer patients. The healing system for cancer patients is adversely affected by the disease. Our immune and healing systems do not function in the same manner as non-cancer individuals. We

lean heavily on the vagaries of the *Goddess of Health*.
Like our non-cancer brothers and sisters we become
targets for all manner of illness. It's just that it is harder
for us to deal with them.

The point to remember is that we traveling on the
Big C have more on our plates than the disease, itself,
on any given day.

*   *   *

Not all of my experiences as a cancer victim involve
pain or discomfort to the body. Every now and then a
touch of humor takes center stage.

The incident that I am now reporting culminated 15
minutes ago.

It all began three days ago. At the time in question,
I was in my living room. I was going outside to move
the garbage receptacle to streetside for the morrow's
pick up. I flicked the porch light on. The light went on
instantly. Then POW!!! It blew out. No doubt about it -
the light bulb was dead.

Removing the bulb, for me, was not an easy given. It
took a lot of effort. A side effect from my chemo is loss
of much feeling in my fingers and hands. I also have
a strength problem (this I am attempting to correct by
exercises at the fitness center). I would say that it took
at least three minutes to unscrew the bulb. In the process
of inserting my hand between the glass shade and the
bulb I nicked the back of my hand. It was caused by the
metal strip portion of the shade. Blood spurted from the
nicks like there was no tomorrow.

NOTE: The dermatologist has since explained that
as we become older the fat goes away from the back

of our hands. It is that fat that protects us from the bleeding that I encountered. (MY CONCLUSION: So, all fat ain't bad)

After negotiating a Band-Aid on my hand I screwed a new bulb into the socket. It is to be noted that I'm 5'8" and the socket is about 13" above my head. At night, with a balance problem and loss of feelings in my fingers and hands it presented a minor problem. In any event, I screwed the bulb in and flicked on the switch. Still no illumination.

Not to be deterred, I secured another bulb and repeated the process - same negative result.

Being a great householder I descended the interior steps to the basement (step climbing and descending is always a problem for me). I checked the breakers - none had tripped.

To me, it became apparent that the switch was shot. Since I didn't smell any burning I ruled out shorts or burned wires or whatevers (I know nothing about electricity).

Knowing my limitations I felt that prudence dictated that I back off and not play at being an electrician.

The next day I telephoned a neighborhood *handyman* who sported a good reputation. I had never met him. I explained my plight. I also discussed with him several long overdue household projects - all safety oriented.

The next day he appeared at my door.

Standing upon the porch as I opened the door was a handsome man in his late 30s. He stood 6'6" tall.

I invited him in and explained my dilemma. That very evening was Halloween, I explained. I had no working porch light. I would be unable to properly accommodate the youngsters that evening.

He agreed.

Still on the porch, he inserted his hand under the bulb and twisted it one time - VOILA! *and there was light!*

No longer do things like that embarrass me. In days of yore it certainly would have. But, for the time being I can use the *crutch* of cancer as my justification for not being able to screw a light bulb into place.

My new friend, L. the *handyman* discussed the other projects that he would undertake.

As he departed, to play it safe, I asked that he not recount the incident of the light bulb to too many people.

Yes, the life of a cancer victim can be sprinkled with laughs.

NOTE: That evening I quickly suspended this writing project. Hurriedly, I threw a frozen dinner into the microwave. Time did not permit me to prepare something more enjoyable. I gobbled my dinner. Then, like my departed wife had trained me to do, I set the sweets by the door.

It was exactly 7 p.m. The trick-or-treaters would soon be here.

It was 8 p.m., and the first was yet to come.

I checked the calendar.

Halloween was not due until the following Friday.

* * *

Now we return to the next regimen of chemotherapy.

Upon completion of the multi cycles of Taxotere I underwent another catscan. The good Dr. G. decided that he would embark upon a new approach. He reasoned, I assume, that if a chemo regimen of Carboplatin was good enough for Lance Armstrong it was good enough for me.

I became very excited about its prospects for success. So much so, that I scurried about to acquaintances *with hat in hand* asking for donations. I was asking for sponsorship for Team Warren Evans which would enter that coming summer's Tour de France. After all, if Carboplatin could cure Lance and make it possible for him to do the bike racing thing why not Warren?

Unfortunately, it was not to be.

The regimen didn't work for me and consequently I could not do the Tour de France thing that next summer.

Just as well - I'm not much for racing bikes up hill.

*   *   *

Not one to give up, the very caring Dr. G. aggressively continued his research on my behalf.

One day he came to me and discussed a possibility that he was trying to hatch. There was a drug called Velcade that had been approved several weeks earlier. If memory serves me right, he said that it had been successfully used in the treatment of Myloma. There was one very disturbing caveat. The cost of the drug was prohibitively high.

It was his intention to contact the pharmaceutical company and plead on my behalf for the drug. The drug had been approved for Myloma treatment and not for Prostate Cancer treatment. Under those circumstances neither Medicare nor the insurance companies would approve it for me. Dr. G. further explained that it would take "weeks or months" before he would hear from the drug company.

In the meantime he was going to try something else on me.

*   *   *

Without further ado, Dr. G. placed me on a new regimen of chemotherapy. The prescription given to me instructed me to take one capsule a day for the two days prior to chemo. I was also to take one on the day of chemo and one a day for the next two days. It would begin that coming weekend.

When the pharmacist finished going over my instructions he hit me with a giant *time bomb.* "Warren," said my heretofore good friend at the pharmacy, "with your co-pay that will be $401.01."

Never in the past had I ever paid such a great amount for a drug. Between Medicare and my insurance company the figures were always small. If not small, they were, at least, manageable. I had no choice but to flash my VISA.

From their safe place in my refrigerator came my weekend ration of capsules. I took them as directed both Saturday and Sunday.

On Monday I reported for my chemo - oops! What I hadn't realized was the fact that the capsules, Etoposide, was a chemo drug in itself. That accounted for the king's ransom that I had to pay for them. That Saturday I had already commenced my chemotherapy regimen. Only the part that I administered was delivered orally.

The Monday installment involved hooking me up to the IV portion of the chemotherapy. The drug that was delivered to my body by IV was called Adreomycin.

From Nurse S., who administered the Adreomycin,

I was to learn something very startling about my new regimen. She explained that I was being given one of the older forms of chemotherapy. Over the years, it has been given primarily to breast cancer patients. She further explained that many regimens of chemotherapy had been supplanted by more advanced formulations. As for the tried and true Adreomycin-Etoposide formulation - it continues to perform its mission. No *magic pill* has taken its place.

Incidentally, to Nurse S. I cried my tale of woe concerning the $401.01 tab that I had to pay.

She shook her head and explained that it should never have been. "Recently," she said, "Medicare's rules were changed. They would now pay for a chemo drug if it could be given by IV - no matter what form of delivery the drug would take. Since Etoposide can be given by IV infusion they would pay for Etoposide if taken orally."

I would later find a phone number in Indianapolis for the office of Medicare that could handle my specific claim. My call to them was very productive.

The following day I contacted the pharmacy and gave them details of my conversation with the Medicare people.

Within a week I had a check for $400 even from the pharmacy. I never said anything about the $1.01.

The regimen was to continue for about three months.

During one of my meets with Dr. G. I complained about the capsules. I told him that they were giving my digestive system a fit.

Chapter 9   *The Tide has Turned*

"IT'S A MIRACLE - IT'S A MIRACLE," D1, the Gatekeeper, kept repeating to me on the phone. "That's what Dr. G kept saying. He said that it was a miracle."

I had just called the cancer clinic to find out if they had received the results on my last catscan. I was supposed to have a meet with Dr. G. when they were received. At that time we would plan the next step. I was unable to get through to him. D1 had fielded my call. She told me that the results had been received and that she would contact Dr. G.

Thirty minutes later she called me at home. She began the conversation with the excited "It's a miracle" refrain.

"Mr. Evans, I did get to speak to Dr. G. When I spoke with him he was so excited. He kept saying 'it's a miracle - miracle - it's a miracle.' He then told me that he was 'so overwhelmed' that he couldn't talk to you now but he would contact you. In the meantime, he dictated the results to me."

From my receiver I could hear the gatekeeper shuffling through pieces of paper. "Excuse me, Mr. Evans, but I'm trying to make sense of the report that Dr. G.

dictated to me. You have to understand …" She didn't finish the sentence. "Anyway, he kept repeating over and over that 'it was a miracle' … now bear with me if I don't have the exact wording … there was a marked improvement in the pulmonary nodules - the nodule in right upper lobe has been resected - others appear to have been diminished in size - none have shown progressive enlargement and no new nodules are detected."

I was unable to understand my notes on her comment regarding the abdomen. I am inclined to think that it was a favorable report. "... abdomen decrease - stable appearance of the mass in right kidney - no new lesions are present."

You must understand that for three years I have been the recipient of radiation and numerous forms of chemotherapy and other treatments. Unfortunately, none have addressed the problem sufficiently to be considered successful.

You can not imagine: How elated I am. Or how thankful I am to Dr. G. for his dogged persistence in trying every imaginable possibility on me. Never did he give up.

I am grateful that my oncologist is dedicated to his patients and that I am numbered amongst them.

He has taken a patient, me, that two years ago he tagged for the undertaker. One that looked like "death" and persisted with one treatment after another. Rather than getting discouraged he just kept trying.

In an earlier chapter I recounted the problems that I had with my personal *plumbing* system. There was a cancerous obstruction within my penis that was very bothersome and necessitated the employment of self catheterization.

I am overjoyed to report that the *miracle* has included this very serious problem.

How fortunate am I to have Dr. G. and the good Lord as teammates, on my side.

Realistically, I must accept the fact that every coin has two sides and there are no guarantees. What may be today's good news can turn bad overnight.

But, I will continue to take each day as it comes and will not *beg trouble.*

In the meantime, I thank God, Dr. G., and the tried and true women's breast cancer chemotherapy regimen consisting of Etoposide and Adreomyacin.

My current regimen consists of the same Etoposide except that it is now given in IV form. I continue to take the Adreomyacin in IV form. This chemo treatment is given to me once every three weeks. The dose of Adreomyacin is larger because of the change in frequency.

It is administered as follows:

Monday - (approx. 2 1/2 hours): Chemo including both Etoposide and Adreomyacin.

Tuesday - (approx. 2 hours) Etoposide in IV form.

Wednesday - (approx. 2 hours) Etoposide in IV form.

Thursday - (5 minutes) Injection of Neulast (for white blood count).

For the next two weeks I have a pass from chemo. I merely check in on Mondays for my bloodwork. Needless to say I continue taking the Procrit for my red count. Incidentally, the Neulast shots address the white count.

Chapter 10   *A Credo for Me*

In reading the previous pages you may wonder why I took the approach that I did. You certainly, after reading those pages, have a perfect right to question my approach.

Simply put, I have tried to share with you virtually EVERYTHING that I have been going through beginning with the diagnosis three years ago to the present.

It is my greatest hope that my report may help, at least, one other fellow cancer victim. Of equal importance is that my story be read by families and personal caregivers of cancer victims. After all, when it's said and done - all of us suffering from cancer need the love, prayers, and care from those that surround us.

If, perchance a medical caregiver should read this it is my sincere wish that my story may give you just one more perspective from the patient side of the examining table.

No two of us are alike. God wanted it that way when he created us. I would guess that all cancer victims have had varying experiences on our voyage with *Big C*. Mine, is just one more.

In this writing I have attempted, by many illustrations, to explain what has brought me to where I am today. I honestly and truly feel that I have a better understanding of myself and the world around me today than I did when it all started.

I believe that I am more of a people person than I ever was before. This, I believe, has made me less self-centered.

It is my hope that I am more tolerant and appreciative of others than I had been in the past.

My philosophy on life is far different than it ever was three years ago. Here are some of the tenets that I now try to live by. (Not necessarily in order).

1. I shall live one day at a time.

2. I will not complain that I wear tight shoes lest I meet a man with no feet at all.

3. There are no guarantees in life.

4. I do not want others to prematurely mourn my passing because I could easily attend their final rites.

5. Keep physically active.

6. Keep mentally active.

7. Keep socially active.

8. Listen to your body - work it sensibly. Monitor it for change but never dwell on lack thereof.

9. Eat and drink sensibly. Keep properly nourished and never allow yourself to become dehydrated or starved.

10. Establish and maintain good sleep habits.

11. Monitor your bodily functions and assure yourself that they function as they should.

12. Do not fail to contact your medical caregiver when there is a problem with your body.

13. Do not fail to contact your non-medical caregiver(s) when you have a personal problem that requires attention.

14. Keep a day by day journal of your health report card and bring it to your next scheduled appointment with your physician.

15. Take notes at meetings with your doctor or have your caregiver do so in your stead.

16. Keep up-to-date on all of your finances. Your mind must always be at rest from financial problems and focused on more important things.

17. Keep as active as you can but do not over do it.

18. Maintain a close relationship with the Supreme Being that you worship.

19. The more activities that you do in concert with others the happier you will be.

20. Focus on today and neither dwell upon the past nor be preoccupied with the future.

21. Follow the regimen prescribed by your medical caregivers.

22. Once 21 above, is accomplished remove your focus from your medical problems. Look for the sunshine of life not the rainfall.

23. Have happy thoughts about people. Do not harbor bad feelings toward anybody. If the latter is not possible than put that individual(s) out of your mind.

24. Smile and greet others that you meet - it's infectious.

25. Love and respect yourself.

26. Do not dwell on what could have been.

27. Live your life within your own limitations. Do not try to meet the standards of others.

28. Enjoy! You deserve it.

29. Pray for others then pray for yourself.

30. *Smile and the world smiles with you - cry and you cry alone.*

31. Do something useful - *It will keep you off the streets.*

32. *Count your blessings - just remember the man that had no foot at all.*

Epilogue

This has been a work of love. For me, the past three years have been an adventure. Each day has been a new experience for me. Some have been very unpleasant and others have been great.

I have no great expectations for myself. I truly believe that I must accept the hand that is dealt me. Whatever is to be, will be. I shall do my best to cooperate in the endeavor to extend my longevity. Beyond that, there is no more that I can do.

It is my hope that you will have enjoyed meeting the people with whom I have been exposed. In your life there are individuals that will have the same importance to you. Get to know and love them. You'll be glad that you did.

This is my hope for this book: *That this book convey at least one thing to one person that will make his/her life a better one.* If it does, than the work that I have expended will have been worth the while.

When my journey began I was embarrassed and ashamed to be a cancer victim. Now, I feel that I am just one more individual that, incidentally, happens to have cancer.

*   *   *

I ran into Dr. B.'s pretty wife, A., the other day. She's a very highly regarded physical therapist. Always ready to *milk* a professional for free advice, I complained to her about a rotator cuff problem.

Along with some exercises, she recommended swimming. When I explained that I had Edema, she became more persistent. The hydrostatic action of the water would be excellent ... "best thing in the world for Edema. Ask Dr. P. for this thoughts."

I saw my dermatologist, Dr. P., and he became ecstatic about what swimming would do for my body - added to that it would be very relaxing. So, now I'll be joining all my friends that swim at the fitness center.

*   *   *

HAPPY TIMING FOR HAPPY NEWS - While sitting at my desk recently, putting the final red marks on the galley for this manuscript, I received an unexpected, but most welcome call from Dr. T., my primary care physician.

He excitedly phoned me with the results of the most recent catscan taken two days earlier. It showed a marked improvement over the one taken three months earlier. That was the one that Dr. G. had referred to as a "miracle."

On the following day, at my scheduled visit with Dr. G., he confirmed the good news. In keeping with his team approach, he asked me what my preference would be at this stage. I countered by suggesting that we temporarily discontinue my chemotherapy regimen if he felt comfortable with that option.

He smiled as he responded. "We will discontinue your chemo pending the results from your next catscan three months from now." He was beaming.

It turned out to be one of the happiest days of my life.

About the Author

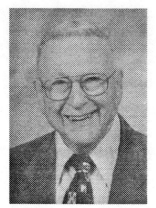

WARREN EVANS, from his beginning as a newspaper writer gravitated into the world of travel. For many of those years he managed to work in both the field of travel and writing.

Among his credits are two travel guides: CHINA-THE RETURN OF MARCO POLO and VIRGINIA-THE WESTERN HIGHLANDS.

His three previously written murder mysteries are: RED LEAF 645, THE CORPSE MOWS AT MID-NIGHT, and MARVELOUS MAGGIE.